The Genetic Mystery of Cold Hands and Feet

A comprehensive guide to understanding, treating, and living with Raynaud's phenomenon, including the latest research breakthroughs and promising therapies.

Callista DeLuca

Copyright © 2024 Callista Deluca.

All rights reserved. Without the publisher's prior written permission, no part of this publication may be reproduced, distributed, or transmitted in any form or by any means, including photocopying, recording, or other electronic or mechanical methods, except for brief quotations embodied in critical reviews and certain other noncommercial uses permitted by copyright law.

Table of Contents

Introduction   **6**
   Understanding Raynaud's phenomenon.   6
   Raynaud's disease and its genetic basis   7
   An Overview of Current Treatments   7

Chapter 1.   **9**
   Unraveling the Genetic Basis of Raynaud's   9
   Journey of Genetic Discovery   9
   Raynaud's disease involves key genes.   11

Chapter 2.   **14**
   Primary Raynaud's: Insights and Management.   14
   Understanding primary Raynaud's.   14
   Lifestyle Modifications to Manage Symptoms   15
   Medications and therapies   16

Chapter 3   **19**
   Secondary Raynaud's Disease: Causes and Complications   19
   Exploring Secondary Raynaud's Phenomenon   19
   Autoimmune diseases and Raynaud's   20
   Complications and challenges.   22

Chapter 4   **24**
   Novel Approaches to Treatment   24
   Targeted Therapies Based on Genetic Information   24
   Promising Drug Developments   25
   Alternative and Complementary Therapies   27

Chapter 5   **30**
   Living well with Raynaud's.   30
   Coping Techniques for Everyday Life   30
   Tips for Managing Symptoms Across Seasons   31

Support Networks and Resources	32
Chapter 6	**34**
Progress in Research and Future Directions	34
Potential Breakthroughs On the Horizon	36
Conclusion	**40**

Introduction

Raynaud's phenomenon, which is defined by bouts of cold-induced vasospasm in the extremities, presents major problems to people affected.

This introduction lays the groundwork for a thorough investigation of Raynaud's disease, giving light on its prevalence, symptoms, and impact on daily life.

By diving into the physiological principles that underpin this illness, readers get insight into the complicated interaction of blood vessels, neurons, and environmental stimuli.

Furthermore, the introduction highlights the significance of comprehending Raynaud's disease not just from a clinical standpoint but also in terms of its larger implications for quality of life and mental health.

Understanding Raynaud's phenomenon.

This section delves deeper into the complexities of Raynaud's phenomenon, explaining its primary and secondary manifestations, occurrence across demographics, and triggering events. Readers receive a thorough grasp of how cold temperatures, mental stress, and other stimuli can trigger vasospastic episodes, resulting in the distinct color changes and feelings reported by Raynaud's patients. This section also investigates the range of symptoms associated with the illness, from minor discomfort to severe pain and tissue damage, emphasizing the variation in presentation and severity among affected individuals.

Raynaud's disease and its genetic basis

Familial clustering and heritability studies show that genetics play a significant role in predisposing people to Raynaud's phenomenon. This section dives into the genetic basis of the illness, examining recent advances in genomic research and identifying important genes involved in its development.

By deciphering the molecular principles driving vascular reactivity and thermoregulation, readers gain insight into why certain people are more prone to vasospastic events.

Furthermore, this part investigates the relationship between genetic predisposition and environmental variables, emphasizing the complex interaction that finally leads to Raynaud's in sensitive individuals.

An Overview of Current Treatments

Managing Raynaud's necessitates a multimodal approach that covers both immediate symptom alleviation and long-term disease control.

This section includes a detailed summary of current treatment options, which range from lifestyle changes and behavioral treatments to pharmaceutical medicines and surgical procedures.

Readers learn about the reasoning behind each therapeutic technique, as well as the possible advantages, limits, and adverse effects associated with various approaches. Furthermore, this part investigates developing therapy techniques and innovative treatment targets based on recent advances in genetic research, providing promise for more successful and tailored approaches to Raynaud's disease management in the future.

Chapter 1.

Unraveling the Genetic Basis of Raynaud's

Understanding the genetic basis of Raynaud's phenomenon is crucial for unraveling its pathophysiology and designing tailored treatment strategies.

This section delves into the history of Raynaud's genetic discoveries, following research from early familial studies to large-scale genome-wide association studies (GWAS).

Researchers have learned more about the molecular mechanisms that cause vasospastic episodes by finding important genes that are linked to the disorder. This makes it possible for personalized therapy and precision medicine to be used in Raynaud's care.

Journey of Genetic Discovery

The search for the genetic basis of Raynaud's phenomenon has been ongoing for several decades, with early studies of familial clustering offering early indications of heritability.

Overall, multidisciplinary approaches, technological advancements, and collaborative efforts have marked the path to genetic discovery in Raynaud's. numbers and restricted genetic technology.

However, when molecular genetics and high-throughput sequencing tools advanced, researchers began to use more systematic methods to find genetic variations related to Raynaud's disease susceptibility.

The introduction of genome-wide association studies (GWAS) allowed researchers to analyze the whole human genome for genetic variations associated with illness risk, marking a watershed moment in Raynaud's genetic research.

GWAS has discovered many susceptibility loci related to Raynaud's disease, offering vital insights into its genetic architecture and pathogenesis.

Furthermore, collaborative initiatives such as multinational consortia and biobanks have made data sharing and meta-analyses easier, allowing researchers to pool resources and discover novel genetic connections with greater statistical power.

In addition to the results from standard GWAS methods, researchers have found rare variants, copy number variations, and regulatory elements that make people more likely to get Raynaud's.

Despite these advances, there are still hurdles to decoding Raynaud's complicated genetic landscape, such as bigger sample numbers, different populations, and functional confirmation of reported genetic variations.

Putting together genetic data with other omics datasets, like transcriptomics and proteomics, could also help us figure out how vasospastic events happen at the molecular level and find new treatment targets.

Overall, multidisciplinary approaches, technological advancements, and collaborative efforts have marked the path to genetic discovery in Raynaud's.

Targeted therapeutics and personalized medicine hold promise for improving outcomes and quality of life for those who suffer from Raynaud's phenomenon as researchers work to understand the genetic basis of the disorder.

Raynaud's disease involves key genes.

Several critical genes have been linked to Raynaud's phenomenon, providing insight into the molecular pathways that underpin vasospastic episodes and vascular dysfunction.

This part looks into how these genes affect the tone of the blood vessels, neurotransmission, and immune response. It does this by giving information on possible therapeutic targets and personalized treatment methods for Raynaud's disease.

One of the genes that has been studied the most in Raynaud's disease is endothelin-1 (EDN1). This gene makes a strong vasoconstrictor peptide that helps control blood flow and vascular tone.

Genetic differences in the EDN1 gene have been linked to a higher risk of Raynaud's phenomenon. This shows how important endothelin-mediated vasoconstriction is in the development of the disease.

Also, differences in genes that make endothelin receptors, like EDNRA and EDNRB, have been linked to a higher risk of getting Raynaud's disease. This shows how important the endothelin pathway is for keeping blood vessels healthy.

The adrenergic receptor gene family, which governs sympathetic nervous system activity and vascular smooth muscle tone, is also an important factor in Raynaud's etiology.

Changes in adrenergic receptor genes, like ADRB2 and ADRB3, have been linked to different vascular reactivity and more vasospastic episodes in people who have Raynaud's.

Also, variations in genes that make neurotransmitter transporters, such as SLC6A2 and SLC6A4, have been linked to incorrect catecholamine signaling and irregular activity of the sympathetic nerve. These things help explain the vasospastic effects seen in Raynaud's.

In addition to genes involved in vascular control, immunological dysregulation plays an important role in the etiology of Raynaud's phenomenon, especially in secondary variants linked with autoimmune disorders.

People who have TNF-α and IL-6 genes are more likely to have autoimmune vasculopathies and endothelial dysfunction, which makes it hard for the body to control blood flow and causes tissue damage.

Also, variations in genes related to autoimmune diseases, like HLA genes and STAT4, have been linked to a higher risk of secondary

Raynaud's. This shows how genetic predisposition and immune dysregulation work together in the development of vasospastic disorders.

Overall, the discovery of essential genes involved in Raynaud's phenomenon provides important insights into the molecular mechanisms that cause vasospastic episodes and vascular dysfunction.

Researchers want to create innovative therapeutic tactics and individualized treatment approaches by targeting these genes and their related pathways in order to enhance results and quality of life for Raynaud's patients.

Chapter 2.

Primary Raynaud's: Insights and Management.

Primary Raynaud's illness is the most prevalent type of Raynaud's phenomenon, accounting for the vast majority of cases.

This section delves further into the features, diagnosis, and therapy of primary Raynaud's disease, with an emphasis on lifestyle changes, pharmaceutical therapies, and other interventions aimed at lowering symptom intensity and increasing quality of life for those affected.

Understanding primary Raynaud's.

The main signs of primary Raynaud's syndrome are pallor, cyanosis, and erythema in the extremities caused by vasospastic episodes that happen when the person is cold or stressed.

Unlike secondary Raynaud's, which is frequently associated with underlying medical illnesses such as autoimmune diseases or connective tissue disorders, primary Raynaud's usually occurs in apparently healthy people who have no underlying systemic pathology.

The specific cause of primary Raynaud's remains unknown, but genetic predisposition, aberrant sympathetic nervous system activity, and vascular hyperreactivity are thought to play important roles in its development.

The typical triphasic color changes seen during vasospastic episodes are part of a clinical history and physical examination used to diagnose primary Raynaud's disease.

Additional diagnostic techniques, including nailfold capillaroscopy and cold provocation testing, may be used to evaluate the vascular architecture and responsiveness of afflicted people.

To tell the difference between primary Raynaud's disease and later variants, a differential diagnosis is needed, since the underlying cause and treatment plan may be very different.

Lifestyle Modifications to Manage Symptoms

Lifestyle changes are an important part of primary Raynaud's care, with the goal of reducing symptom triggers, promoting vascular health, and improving afflicted people's cold tolerance.

This section looks at several lifestyle therapies and behavioral methods that can help reduce symptom intensity and frequency, allowing people to better manage their illness on a daily basis.

One of the most effective lifestyle changes for primary Raynaud's is temperature regulation, which entails avoiding cold exposure and keeping the extremities warm by layering clothing, wearing insulated gloves and socks, and using heated blankets or hand warmers in cold environments.

Furthermore, stress management approaches, including relaxation exercises, deep breathing, and mindfulness meditation, might assist in lowering sympathetic nervous system activity and emotional triggers for vasospasm episodes.

Dietary changes may also play a part in primary Raynaud's disease management, since some foods and beverages are thought to worsen symptoms in sensitive individuals.

Caffeine and nicotine-containing goods, for example, might constrict blood vessels and increase vasospastic episodes, whereas diets high in antioxidants and omega-3 fatty acids may have vasodilatory and anti-inflammatory properties, thus lowering symptom intensity in certain people.

Regular physical exercise is another critical component of primary Raynaud's therapy since it promotes cardiovascular health, increases circulation, and improves overall vascular function.

Low-impact workouts like walking, swimming, and cycling can help boost peripheral blood flow and reduce the frequency of vasospastic events, while also improving mood, stress reduction, and general well-being.

Medications and therapies

In addition to lifestyle changes, pharmaceutical therapy and other interventions may be indicated for people with primary Raynaud's disease, especially those who have severe or refractory symptoms that interfere with everyday activities.

This section examines the various drugs and treatments available for primary Raynaud's management, focusing on their mechanisms of action, effectiveness, and potential adverse effects.

Calcium channel blockers (CCBs) are the first-choice drugs for treating primary Raynaud's disease because they relax the smooth muscle of the blood vessels and improve blood flow to the extremities by stopping calcium from entering cells.

Commonly given CCBs include nifedipine, amlodipine, and diltiazem, which have been found to lessen the incidence and severity of vasospastic events in many people. However, CCBs may cause adverse effects such as headache, dizziness, flushing, and peripheral edema, limiting their acceptability and long-term usage in some individuals.

As extra treatment for primary Raynaud's disease, other vasodilatory drugs like alpha-blockers, angiotensin-converting enzyme (ACE) inhibitors, and phosphodiesterase inhibitors may be looked into. This is especially true for people who do not respond well to CCBs or who cannot use them because of a health problem.

Topical nitroglycerin ointment or patches can also be given to afflicted extremities during acute vasospastic episodes to enhance vasodilation and relieve symptoms.

People whose symptoms are severe or do not go away may be given more invasive treatments, like digital sympathectomy or botulinum toxin injections, to stop sympathetic nerve activity and lessen vasospastic episodes.

However, these procedures are normally reserved for instances that are recalcitrant to conservative therapy and need a comprehensive assessment of possible risks and benefits.

Non-pharmacological therapy, including biofeedback training, acupuncture, and transcutaneous electrical nerve stimulation (TENS), may also provide symptomatic relief for some people with primary Raynaud's disease; however, evidence for their effectiveness is limited. Furthermore, lifestyle changes and behavioral treatments should remain the foundation of primary Raynaud's disease management, with pharmaceutical therapy and other interventions adapted to individual requirements and preferences in conjunction with a healthcare physician.

Overall, primary Raynaud's care necessitates a complex strategy that includes both immediate symptom alleviation and long-term disease management, with a focus on lifestyle changes, pharmaceutical therapies, and other interventions suited to individual requirements and preferences. Healthcare practitioners can enhance quality of life and functional results for those suffering from primary Raynaud's by enabling them to better manage their illness and reduce symptom load.

Chapter 3

Secondary Raynaud's Disease: Causes and Complications

Secondary Raynaud's phenomenon, also known as Raynaud's syndrome, is the result of an underlying medical disease or external stimulus that causes vasospastic episodes in the limbs.

This section delves further into secondary Raynaud's illness, including its genesis, related conditions, probable consequences, and diagnostic and treatment issues.

Exploring Secondary Raynaud's Phenomenon

Secondary Raynaud's phenomenon is defined by vasospastic episodes caused by underlying medical problems, drugs, or environmental factors. Secondary Raynaud's is frequently connected with systemic conditions such as autoimmune disorders, connective tissue diseases, and vascular abnormalities, as opposed to primary Raynaud's, which usually affects otherwise healthy people.

Furthermore, some drugs, occupational exposures, and lifestyle choices may worsen or induce vasospastic episodes in vulnerable people.

The association of secondary Raynaud's with particular underlying illnesses or disorders can provide useful information about its cause and management. Systemic sclerosis (scleroderma), systemic lupus erythematosus (lupus), rheumatoid arthritis, Sjögren's syndrome, and dermatomyositis are some of the most common underlying disorders associated with secondary Raynaud's.

People who are more likely to get vasospastic episodes may also be exposed to vibrating tools at work, develop hand-arm vibration syndrome (HAVS), or take certain drugs, like beta-blockers, ergotamine derivatives, and chemotherapeutic agents.

Understanding the underlying etiology of secondary Raynaud's is critical for making informed diagnostic and therapeutic decisions. Clinicians must undertake a complete medical history, physical examination, and laboratory testing to identify probable underlying disorders or triggers and distinguish secondary Raynaud's from the main forms of the condition.

To find out more about a patient's vascular morphology, immunological function, and underlying disease, diagnostic methods like nailfold capillaroscopy, autoimmune serology, imaging exams, and vascular testing can be used.

Autoimmune diseases and Raynaud's

Autoimmune diseases are a major group of underlying diseases connected with secondary Raynaud's phenomenon. This shows how immune dysregulation and vascular dysfunction are intricately linked in their development.

This part looks into how autoimmune diseases and Raynaud's are connected, focusing on systemic sclerosis (also called scleroderma), systemic lupus erythematosus (also called lupus), and other connective tissue disorders that are often connected with secondary Raynaud's.

Systemic sclerosis (SSc), also referred to as scleroderma, is a chronic autoimmune condition that manifests as extensive fibrosis and vascular abnormalities like Raynaud's phenomenon. The characteristic of SSc-related Raynaud's is its early start, severe course, and progressive nature, which frequently results in digital ulcers, gangrene, and tissue necrosis in afflicted patients. Endothelial function issues, microvascular damage, and improper immunological responses are the causes of Raynaud's in SSc. This makes it hard to control blood flow and causes tissue ischemia in the limbs.

Systemic lupus erythematosus (SLE), often known as lupus, is another autoimmune condition that is frequently linked to secondary Raynaud's phenomenon, particularly in individuals who have active disease and circulating autoantibodies. Raynaud's disease in SLE may be an early sign of vascular inflammation and immune complex deposition before additional systemic symptoms such as arthritis, rash, and kidney involvement. Other diseases affecting connective tissues, like rheumatoid arthritis, Sjogren's syndrome, and dermatomyositis, can show up as secondary Raynaud's. This shows the wide range of autoimmune diseases that can cause vasospastic symptoms.

Complications and challenges.

Secondary Raynaud's phenomenon is more likely to cause problems and consequences than primary forms of the syndrome. This is because of its cause, severity, and related conditions.

This section investigates the potential complications and challenges in the diagnosis and management of secondary Raynaud's disease, emphasizing the importance of early detection, multidisciplinary care, and targeted interventions to reduce negative outcomes and improve quality of life for those affected.

One of the most serious symptoms of secondary Raynaud's is digital ischemia, which can cause digital ulcers, gangrene, or tissue necrosis in extreme instances. Vasospastic events that last a long time and happen again and again can lead to chronic tissue hypoxia, endothelial damage, and slow wound healing in patients, which can lead to digital ulceration and tissue loss.

If you do not treat secondary Raynaud's syndrome that is linked to autoimmune diseases like systemic sclerosis (SSc), it can get worse and lead to scleroderma renal crises, pulmonary arterial hypertension, and other life-threatening problems.

Secondary Raynaud's syndrome can be difficult to diagnose because of its complex origin, overlapping symptoms, and varying presentation across underlying conditions. Clinicians must perform a thorough assessment, including a medical history, physical examination, laboratory tests, and imaging scans, to identify probable triggers or underlying problems that contribute to vasospastic episodes.

A differential diagnosis is required to differentiate secondary Raynaud's from the main types of the disorder and begin appropriate therapy based on the underlying pathology and disease severity.

Secondary Raynaud's needs a multidisciplinary approach that addresses both the underlying disease activity and vasospastic symptoms, along with personalized therapies that are based on each person's needs and preferences. Pharmacological therapy such as calcium channel blockers, vasodilators, and immunosuppressive drugs may be used to treat vasospastic episodes and reduce autoimmune inflammation.

In addition, non-pharmacological therapies such as lifestyle changes, vocational adaptations, and digital security measures may help reduce symptom intensity and avoid problems in afflicted individuals.

Overall, secondary Raynaud's phenomenon presents unique problems and complications in diagnosis and care, necessitating a collaborative and tailored approach to improve results and quality of life for those affected. Healthcare professionals can successfully limit the effects of secondary Raynaud's by treating underlying disease activity, controlling vasospastic symptoms, and reducing risk factors for complications.

Chapter 4

Novel Approaches to Treatment

In recent years, advances in understanding the genetic basis of Raynaud's phenomenon have led to the development of innovative therapeutic options. This section delves into the most recent advances in targeted therapy based on genetic discoveries, prospective medication advancements, and alternative and complementary medicines for treating Raynaud's phenomenon.

Researchers want to improve symptom management, improve quality of life, and lessen the impact of this severe disorder on afflicted people by using genetic knowledge and investigating novel treatment methods.

Targeted Therapies Based on Genetic Information

One of the most promising approaches to treating Raynaud's phenomenon is the creation of tailored treatments based on genetic information.

By identifying critical genes and molecular pathways involved in the condition's etiology, researchers can pinpoint possible treatment targets and develop precision medications for particular patients.

For instance, genetic studies have found genes that could be used to treat Raynaud's disease. These genes are involved in neurotransmitter signaling pathways, vascular tone modulation, and endothelial function.

Researchers want to fix vascular homeostasis, lower vasospastic episodes, and improve peripheral blood flow in people who have these issues by changing these pathways with targeted therapies such as small-molecule inhibitors, monoclonal antibodies, or gene editing technologies.

Furthermore, advances in personalized medicine and pharmacogenomics allow for the identification of genetic biomarkers that predict therapy responses and the optimization of therapeutic regimens for particular individuals.

Clinicians can adjust treatment methods for afflicted people by stratifying them based on their genetic profile and illness subtype.

Promising Drug Developments

In addition to targeted medicines, continuing drug research initiatives show promise for broadening the therapeutic options for Raynaud's phenomenon. Pharmaceutical corporations and university research organizations are actively looking for new therapeutic candidates and repurposing current drugs with potential efficacy in treating vasospastic symptoms and enhancing peripheral circulation.

This is a new kind of possible medicine that works by blocking endothelin, a strong vasoconstrictor peptide that is thought to be connected to Raynaud's.

These medicines enhance vasodilation, improve blood flow, and reduce vasospastic episodes in afflicted patients by blocking endothelin signaling. Clinical trials examining the efficacy and safety of endothelin receptor antagonists in Raynaud's disease are now underway, with preliminary results indicating positive outcomes in specific patient groups.

Researchers are also investigating the therapeutic potential of new vasodilators, anti-inflammatory medicines, and neuroregulatory medications for treating Raynaud's phenomenon. These possible treatments aim to ease symptoms, prevent digital ischemia, and improve patients' quality of life by focusing on important molecular pathways involved in immune system dysregulation, vascular dysfunction, and sympathetic nervous system activity.

Furthermore, repurposing existing pharmaceuticals with vasodilatory, anti-inflammatory, or immunomodulatory qualities is a less expensive and faster way to create Raynaud's drugs.

Preclinical and clinical research has shown that some antidepressants, phosphodiesterase inhibitors, and angiotensin-converting enzyme inhibitors may help treat vasospastic symptoms and improve blood flow to the extremities in Raynaud's disease.

Alternative and Complementary Therapies

Alternative and complementary therapies, in addition to standard pharmaceutical treatments, may provide additional advantages to people suffering from Raynaud's phenomenon.

These treatments, which include acupuncture, herbal medicine, nutritional supplements, and mind-body practices, seek to increase relaxation, enhance circulation, and reduce stress, therefore supplementing traditional therapeutic methods and improving general well-being.

Acupuncture, a traditional Chinese medical procedure that involves inserting small needles into particular acupoints on the body, has been investigated for its possible effectiveness in treating Raynaud's symptoms.

According to a preliminary study, acupuncture may help enhance peripheral blood flow, lower the frequency and intensity of vasospastic episodes, and relieve accompanying symptoms such as pain and numbness in afflicted patients.

However, more well-designed clinical trials are required to determine the safety and efficacy of acupuncture as a supplemental therapy for Raynaud's disease.

Herbal medicine and nutritional supplements, such as Ginkgo biloba, fish oil, and magnesium, have also been studied for their possible vasodilatory and anti-inflammatory properties in Raynaud's phenomenon.

While some studies show that these supplements can help reduce vasospastic symptoms and improve peripheral circulation, evidence for their effectiveness is limited and inconsistent.

Furthermore, safety considerations and potential medication interactions should be considered when utilizing herbal therapies and supplements in combination with traditional Raynaud's therapy.

Mind-body techniques like yoga, meditation, and biofeedback training may also help people with Raynaud's by encouraging relaxation, lowering tension, and modifying autonomic nervous system activity.

These practices focus on mindfulness, deep breathing, and stress reduction strategies, which have been proven to enhance peripheral blood flow, lower sympathetic nervous system activity, and relieve vasospastic episodes in certain Raynaud's patients.

Incorporating mind-body activities into comprehensive treatment regimens may improve symptom management, coping abilities, and overall quality of life for patients.

Alternative and complementary therapies provide potential supplementary ways of controlling Raynaud's phenomenon, complementing traditional treatments, and addressing the condition's complex character.

Researchers want to broaden the therapy armamentarium for Raynaud's by using genetic knowledge and investigating novel treatment methods. Ongoing research initiatives in medication development, personalized medicine, and integrative medicine show promise for advancing the field and improving results for Raynaud's patients.

Chapter 5

Living well with Raynaud's.

Living with Raynaud's phenomenon can be difficult, but with the correct tactics and assistance, people can successfully manage their symptoms and retain a high quality of life. This section delves into coping methods for everyday life, recommendations for managing symptoms in different seasons, and the role of support networks and resources in helping Raynaud's patients to live well and prosper despite their disease.

Coping Techniques for Everyday Life

Managing Raynaud's phenomenon necessitates a proactive strategy that includes lifestyle changes, stress management techniques, and practical ways to reduce symptom triggers and pain.

Coping techniques for everyday life include:

1. **Temperature regulation:** Layering clothing, wearing insulated gloves and stockings, and utilizing heated blankets or hand warmers might help you stay warm and avoid vasospastic episodes caused by cold exposure.

2. **Stress management:** Relaxation techniques such as deep breathing, meditation, and mindfulness can help lower sympathetic nervous system activity and emotional triggers for vasospasm episodes.

3. **Avoiding triggers:** Identifying and avoiding possible triggers such as cold weather, emotional stress, and tobacco smoking might help reduce the frequency and severity of vasospastic episodes in vulnerable people.

4. **Hand and foot care:** Keeping the hands and feet safe from harm, avoiding tight-fitting footwear, and moisturizing the skin on a regular basis will help prevent digital ulcers, fissures, and other Raynaud's consequences.

5. **Regular physical exercise**, such as walking, swimming, or yoga, can improve circulation, reduce stress, and improve overall vascular health in people with Raynaud's disease.

6. **Occupational adjustments:** Making ergonomic changes in the workplace, utilizing vibration-dampening instruments, and taking regular pauses to warm up might help reduce occupational exposures and prevent Raynaud's symptoms from worsening.

Tips for Managing Symptoms Across Seasons

Raynaud's symptoms may fluctuate with variations in temperature and meteorological conditions, necessitating that patients adjust their care options accordingly.

1. **Winter**: Dressing warmly in insulated clothes, wearing gloves and stockings at all times, and utilizing heated attachments like hand warmers or heated steering wheels might help reduce cold-induced vasospasm in the winter.

2. **Summer:** To reduce vasospastic episodes caused by heat or sun exposure, avoid using excessive air conditioning, apply sun protection to prevent sunburn on exposed skin, and remain hydrated to maintain appropriate blood flow.

3. **Transitional seasons**: Gradually acclimating to temperature changes, layering clothes to accommodate for temperature swings, and being aware of rapid weather changes can all help people manage Raynaud's symptoms in transitional seasons like spring and fall.

4. **Travel:** Planning ahead of time for trips to colder or warmer areas, carrying suitable clothes and accessories, and taking breaks to warm up or cool down as required can help Raynaud's patients enjoy their travels while limiting symptom exacerbations.

Support Networks and Resources

Individuals living with Raynaud's phenomenon might greatly benefit from developing a strong support network and having access to reputable services.

Support networks and resources, including:

1. Patient advocacy groups, such as the Raynaud's Association and the Scleroderma Foundation, offer information, support, and resources to

those living with Raynaud's and similar disorders, such as online forums, educational materials, and community activities.

2. Open communication with healthcare professionals, such as primary care physicians, rheumatologists, and vascular specialists, can assist clients in receiving comprehensive care, tailored treatment suggestions, and continuous support for Raynaud's disease management.

3. Joining a local or online support group for people with Raynaud's disease can provide opportunities for peer support, shared experiences, and practical ideas for dealing with the problems of the condition.

4. Educational materials: Having access to reliable educational materials, books, articles, and online resources about Raynaud's phenomenon can help people gain a better understanding of the condition, learn management strategies, and stay up-to-date on the latest research and developments.

Individuals with Raynaud's disease can effectively manage their symptoms, improve their quality of life, and live well despite the obstacles presented by their illness by implementing coping methods for everyday life, adjusting to seasonal changes, and gaining access to support networks and resources.

Chapter 6

Progress in Research and Future Directions

Recent developments in research have given insight into the underlying processes of Raynaud's phenomenon, opening the door to novel therapeutic methods and targeted medicines. Cutting-edge Raynaud's research spans several fields, including genetics, vascular biology, immunology, and neuroscience, with the goal of understanding the intricate interaction of elements that contribute to vasospastic episodes and tissue ischemia in afflicted individuals.

Genetic studies have revealed critical genes and molecular pathways involved in Raynaud's pathogenesis, shedding light on the condition's heritability and prospective therapeutic targets. Genome-wide association studies (GWAS) have found genetic variations connected to Raynaud's risk and severity. This shows how important vascular tone modulation, endothelial dysfunction, and neurovascular communication are to the disease's cause.

Researchers want to create individualized therapy options for Raynaud's disease based on individual patients' genetic profiles and disease subtypes.

Advances in vascular biology have revealed new pathways that underpin vasospastic events and tissue ischemia in Raynaud's.
Endothelial dysfunction, microvascular abnormalities, and vasoactive mediators that are not working right all play major roles in patients who have trouble controlling blood flow and getting enough oxygen to their tissues.

Researchers want to create tailored therapeutics to restore vascular homeostasis and reduce vasospastic symptoms in Raynaud's disease by better understanding the molecular processes underlying vascular tone regulation and endothelial function.

Studies on the immune system have shown that autoimmune dysregulation and inflammatory mediators are involved in the development of secondary Raynaud's phenomenon. This is especially true for individuals who already have autoimmune diseases such as systemic sclerosis (scleroderma) or systemic lupus erythematosus (lupus).
People who have this condition have vascular inflammation, endothelial damage, and tissue fibrosis because their immune systems are not working right. Making autoantibodies and depositing immune complexes are the causes of this.

Researchers want to uncover immunomodulatory targets and create innovative treatment techniques to decrease autoimmune inflammation and avoid tissue damage in Raynaud's patients by better understanding the immunopathogenesis.

According to neurobiological studies, issues with the sympathetic nervous system and the control of nerves and blood vessels are what cause Raynaud's phenomenon. This shows how important autonomic dysfunction is in vasospastic episodes and digital ischemia.

Altered neurotransmitter release, sympathetic hyperactivity, and peripheral nerve dysfunction all lead to excessive vasoconstriction and poor blood flow control in afflicted people.

Researchers want to create neuroprotective medicines, neuromodulatory treatments, and biofeedback techniques to modify autonomic tone and enhance peripheral circulation in afflicted patients by better understanding the neurobiological underpinnings underlying Raynaud's disease.

Potential Breakthroughs On the Horizon

Looking ahead, numerous possible discoveries show promise for furthering Raynaud's research and altering clinical care for afflicted people. This includes:

Genetically targeted therapies: Personalized therapy techniques tailored to specific patients' genetic profiles and disease subtypes have the potential to enhance treatment results and minimize the burden of Raynaud's symptoms.

Researchers want to make precise therapies that target specific genes and molecular pathways involved in the cause of Raynaud's disease in order to restore vascular homeostasis, reduce vasospastic symptoms, and stop tissue damage in patients.

Ongoing medication development efforts are aimed at discovering new vasodilators, anti-inflammatory medicines, and neuroregulatory therapies that may be effective in treating Raynaud's phenomenon. Researchers want to broaden Raynaud's therapy arsenal by investigating novel pharmacological targets and repurposing existing drugs, providing more effective therapeutic alternatives for those affected. Emerging therapeutic techniques, including gene therapy, cell-based treatments, and tissue engineering, have the potential to restore vascular function and promote tissue healing in Raynaud's.

Researchers want to discover innovative techniques for restoring damaged blood vessels, boosting tissue perfusion, and promoting wound healing in afflicted people by utilizing the regenerative abilities of stem cells, growth factors, and tissue-engineered constructions.

Multidisciplinary approaches: Collaboration among physicians, scientists, engineers, and industry partners is critical for converting research results into clinical applications and improving the area of Raynaud's study.

Researchers want to speed up discovery, create novel treatment techniques, and enhance results for those suffering from Raynaud's phenomenon by encouraging multidisciplinary cooperation and knowledge exchange.

Advances in research and future initiatives have the potential to revolutionize the landscape of Raynaud's care, providing fresh hope for patients and opening the path for individualized, targeted, and creative treatment options.

By leveraging the scientific community's joint efforts, we may continue to solve the secrets of Raynaud's phenomenon and create viable therapeutics to enhance the lives of millions of people living with this condition.

Conclusion

In conclusion, Raynaud's phenomenon is a vascular condition that causes color changes, discomfort, and numbness in the limbs as a result of vasospastic episodes in response to cold or stress.

Recent research has shown the genetic basis of the illness, identified critical genes and pathways, and investigated innovative therapeutic options.

Primary Raynaud's disease is more frequent and controllable, but it generally necessitates lifestyle changes and periodic treatment. Secondary Raynaud's, which is related to underlying illnesses such as autoimmune disorders, needs more extensive treatment.

Coping methods, seasonal adaptations, and support networks all play important roles in helping people live well with Raynaud's.

Advances in genetics, vascular biology, and immunology present exciting opportunities for individualized medicines and targeted interventions.

Innovative therapies, breakthrough medication discoveries, and interdisciplinary methods show promise for increasing symptom management, improving quality of life, and eventually curing Raynaud's phenomenon.

We may work toward better knowledge, management, and outcomes for those impacted by this illness via ongoing research and collaborative activities.

www.ingramcontent.com/pod-product-compliance
Lightning Source LLC
Chambersburg PA
CBHW070951220526
45471CB00007B/2986